PAVING THE WAY

Davina Green

authorHOUSE®

AuthorHouse™ UK Ltd.
500 Avebury Boulevard
Central Milton Keynes, MK9 2BE
www.authorhouse.co.uk
Phone: 08001974150

First published by AuthorHouse 8/13/2009

ISBN: 978-1-4490-1007-2 (sc)

This book is printed on acid-free paper.

DEDICATION

For Joe, Nick and Tim your youthful insights are awesome.

Acknowledgements

I would like to express huge thanks to my Oracle who has patiently listened to me debating with her and myself the various concepts of the book. You have always been my heroine.

To Dr Julie Hare your faith in my endeavours have been heart warming thank you. I appreciate the time that you have devoted to this project and the insightful contributions that you have made, including the prevention of one or two significant typo's.!!

To Karen, Stephanie and your family's my thanks for taking time in your busy lives' to read and share your observations.

To George thank you for your boundless enthusiasm and support.

To Sasha Lee at AuthourHouse, my Publishing Advisor I have appreciated your clear and informative support and your work ethos.

To Claire Price, not quite your name in lights but close to it, my thanks for your illustrations and excellent interpretation of what I wanted portrayed.

To Joe Llewellyn-Jones last but never least, for the front cover, it is beautiful.

The beauty of having children is when they

become a help to you, so Joe Nick and Tim thank you for all your help with copying, pasting, uploading, downloading and scanning, and maybe now tea will be on time.

My warmest thanks to Shirley Curran for letting me reproduce her poem 'Song for 2008', also to The Oldie magazine for granting permission to reproduce. Shirley your support has been much appreciated.

To the team at AuthorHouse, I am indebted to you all for seeing my endeavour reach fruition in this first book.

FOREWORD

What a privilege this is to write for Davina's Carers Companion series of books, and to be part of her journey in seeing her vision for her books coming to fruition in this first edition.

Davina intends this series to be exactly as she names it, a companion for carers. She offers her thoughts, knowledge, tips and advice about various carer issues, drawing from her wealth of experience of sharing the highs and lows, tears and laughter of many carers she has supported over the years. She writes in such a way that carers can dip into topics of interest to them and their situation over time, rather than having to read each book from start to finish. In this way, Davina's vision and hope for this series is to provide easily accessible information, understanding and support to carers in a timely and manageable fashion over the whole course of their caring experience.

Having seen Davina standing alongside carers in many situations, in all stages of illness and in both good and bad times, I can certainly vouch for her being just the right person to write such a series.Indeed, knowing Davina and her work I expect that the beauty of this series will be in her approach; an honest, down to earth style, non-threatening, practical, compassionate, warm, and determined with a generous dose of good fun and humour.

Just as Davina in real life has made a real difference to the carers she has supported, I hope her hard work, and dedication, sincerity, vision and care put into this series of books will also provide just what is needed for whoever dips into these pages. This Carer Companion book series will certainly be a welcome addition to the books I keep close to hand on my own shelves.

By Dr Julie Hare Chartered Clinical Psychologist.

CARING

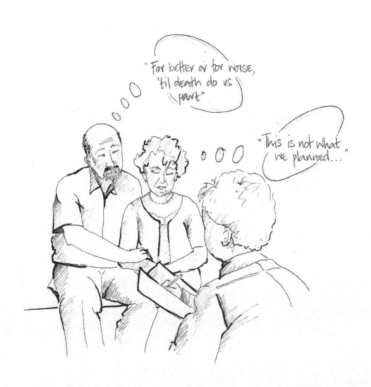

INTRODUCTION

Caring is both proactive and reactive; and without a shadow of a doubt emotional. When I say proactive I mean it is when you feel that you have positive elements of control, often due to accessing timely information leading to knowledge, using your previous experiences, practical help as well as compassionate support. By reactive I refer to the human quality of "knee jerk" responses often caused by exasperation, tiredness and grief. It is emotional because you care.

This book is my small attempt at reducing some of the negative responses and turning them into the more positive elements. Only you and yours can be the judges as to my success. Paving the Way is aimed at unpaid carers of someone with a memory problem. It is not a guide or a manual to caring, as with dieting I fear that if you are unable to achieve something with the frequency you set yourself then you experience a sense of failure. I do not promote failure as I believe each and every one of us can only do the best we are able to; within the boundaries of the information, energy and wellbeing we have at that given moment in time.

This book is intended as a carer's companion,

for you to be able to dip in and out of in spare moments of time and offer some possible options to consider before finalising a decision.

Most importantly if you have any concerns regarding your own memory or that of a loved one do not delay, make an appointment to see your G.P and discuss your worries and observations. There are numerous possible causes for memory problems, not all are a dementia.

The anecdotal content has been amassed over many years working with families who care for someone with a memory problem and is by no means intended as a bible in how to care. It is offered as a collection of explained ideas for your consideration. Hopefully you may find some thought provoking ideas that can be adapted to your circumstances. Without many families allowing me the privilege of sharing their journey this book would not have been possible. To you all I am in your debt.

A SONG FOR 2008

(Sing to the tune of All Things Bright and
Beautiful)

Pension cuts and sheltered homes,
All problems great and small,
Night cramps and insomnia;
We'll overcome them all.
Each bout of acid reflux,
Arthritis that age brings,
The horror of dementia
When we're forgetting things.
The onset of Alzheimer's,
Our fast receding hair,
The fear we'll need to buy a lift
To mount the lofty stair.
All limbs stiff and varicose,
All problems great and small;
Two oh oh eight will be the year
We'll overcome them all.

By Shirley Curran. Gex. France. Printed in Oldie
Magazine. Issue 226 .Jan 2008

THE CARING ROLE

*"It takes less time to do something right
than to explain why
you did them wrong"*

By Henry Wadsworth Longfellow.

Hello. Are you sitting there a little like a startled rabbit in the headlights? Are you quietly wondering at what point you became a carer? Let me hold you by the hand and see if we can work through the bombshell.

You might be surprised to know that you have more skills than you first thought. These skills may be a little rusty and may not have been consciously used for a while but your greatest asset is in knowing the person with a memory problem. Already subtle changes may have begun as unbeknown to you both you have started to make some adjustments.

I guess it may have been your doctor or the Consultant at a Memory Clinic that first referred to you as a carer. Quite possibly it did not initially register but slowly crept over you. Now doubt you secretly look at the person affected and think to yourself...but they look the same. It's not too bad. Nothing has changed. Understandably you maybe

6

resistive to the title Carer, or perhaps crying inside "Why me, Why us? What did we do to deserve this?"

The dementias are a mixed bag of uncontrollable interlopers who move into your life uninvited, they take up residence when you least expect and refuse to move out. A wild range of emotions are often experienced by the carer at this point. The range swings from anger to resignation and back again. With allsorts inbetween.This is normal. As the dawning of a new reality invades your life it is common to experience a grief loss reaction. What makes it harder is if the person....your loved one is aware of the diagnosis and understandably they are also experiencing mixed emotions. The other side of the coin being if the person is unaware of their memory problem, you may feel lonely, isolated and scared for the future. It is not uncommon to find this period of time very difficult. Talking does help for both of you and it can be most positive to talk outside of the family to someone who is not emotionally involved, as well as talking to each other, if you would normally do so. If you do not normally discuss this type of matter with each other it could be a huge jolt. It may be that the person with the memory problem feels that their nose is being rubbed in the open wound of their failings. It is possible that one of you really wants to talk whilst the other just clams up. It is also unlikely that you will both adjust to the diagnosis at the same time. You may both be running an obstacle race but the way you each look at each obstacle is probably not going to be the same.

You may find that the person with the diagnosis feels a wave of relief to have a cause for their memory problem. It is quite possible they feared they were "losing their mind" and despite the nature of the progressive degenerative condition it is better facing the devil with a name, than the devil without a name. We all need to be allowed the right to process new information at our own pace. Despite the diagnosis and unlike many other traumatic situations they can put their house in order, with your help, that of the family and professionals too. It is also possible that they might become introvert for a while as they process, within the limitations of the condition what is taking place. Should you have concerns and feel that they are uncommonly down then go back to the doctor and discuss your observations. It is important to not put everything down to the memory problem, after the entire person is still very much present, although possibly not so easy to reach.

We have all experienced when we have worries how in the small wee hours of the night or when we think no one is watching, that the demons that are our fears unleash themselves and make us appear to behave out of character. Maybe now, gradually over a period of time you will grow to realise odd things that took place over the past couple of years that can now be firmly attributed to the condition. Somehow we gain 20/20 vision in hindsight.

Carers often want to know how to tell if they are

getting it right. The short answer is to be guided by the behaviour and reactions of the person with a memory problem. If they are unwell or unhappy it will translate in the way the respond to life. By the same token if they are well and more or less themselves then in the main all is O.K.

It is without doubt a demanding role you find yourself faced with. The good news is that it is not all doom and gloom. The reason it initially can appear so daunting is because you have not had a job interview. There is no job description. There are no terms of reference. In your working life you had a boss or line manager to check on your performance. You also had your work colleagues who you subconsciously measured yourself against. In this situation you are cast adrift. Without you realising it you have already taken steps of adjusting. Much like being a parent, or starting a new job it is a work in progress and some parts will go more smoothly than others. There will also be good times when the demons are quiet. It depends on the cause of the memory problem as to how the journey will pan out but there are many common issues and emotions.

The response of a new carer varies, some will want all the information they can lay their hands and then possibly struggle with feelings of being overwhelmed by it all, or feel more in control. Some will select an organisation such as The Alzheimer's Society for their specialist support and knowledge as well as a range of services like lunch clubs, support groups, drop- in café's and written material. Each branch delivers their service within their resources. Some people may have other significant medical conditions like Diabetes, Parkinson's disease, Prostrate Problems, and Cancer in fact any of the wide range of illnesses that befall the human being, what ever else that may be going one there is a wealth of associated groups and organisations available. Whichever way you move forward it will not always be at your pace. It may be that you have already been involved in the care of a parent with a memory problem and now are faced with your partner being affected. In this situation it is important to remember that each person in our lives generates a different emotional bond and therefore coping requires different approaches and responses. We are all unique individuals and react to our lot in our own individual way.

HELP

The man who deals in sunshine
Always wins the crowds,
He does far more business
Than the man who peddles clouds.

From the Mormon scriptures (Joy)

Help is an emotive word that conjures up all sorts of images in our minds, for example it would really help if I won the lottery with many fanciful thoughts on what each of us would do with the bountiful amounts of ready cash. The reality is that each of us has an opinion of how much we would like to win. Too much might be a headache to deal with and too little leave us feeling disappointed with our lot," if only it was more...."

Help is very much the same. We have all experienced a situation whereby we have been grateful to a thoughtful unexpected gesture, but we have also known the feeling of being let down, maybe, having been promised grandiose offers that have fallen short of expectation.

Expectation is I believe the key factor to the resulting disappointment, for both the person giving and person receiving help.

Help is a very tricky thing to get right for both

the giver and recipient with many pitfalls along the way. How does the giver know that they will clear the pitfalls with total success? Is total success a reality? A lot of information is needed about the likes and dislikes of the recipient, along with being able to get the timing right whilst ensuring they do not offend or worst still.....find themselves obliged to repeat what was actually a one off offer! In some ways it is short of a miracle that people help each other.

For the recipient there can be pangs of silent, non confessed annoyance or interference which can lead to barriers of offers of help being made when most needed further down the line on the caring journey. Timeliness is paramount and this needs honesty in our communication with those around us. When you are a carer especially of a person with a memory problem all parties need to feel good about what and when and in what format help is accepted. By open and honest communication the boundaries of expectation are declared and all involved are in with a chance of being more satisfied, more often.

I have visited numerous families where I have been told of children living near and far who lead busy lives and have their own family and work life to juggle. No matter how old we are we never stop trying to protect our children from the unpleasant things in life. By doing this we can inadvertently alienate our children from feeling able to reach out to you their parents and be supportive.

The children I have spoken to of these same

parents have often relayed to me how either Mum or Dad are proud or private people who would not accept anything. A deadlock exists by default. Talking together can positively enable all parties. For example by finding out that either Mum or Dad is managing o.k. ....but misses meeting with friends can be liberating as this allows offers to be made of sitting with the person who has a memory problem allowing the other parent a few much needed hours of respite.

The opportunity of parent sitting can open a window to the child into what it is like to care for a person with a memory problem 24/7 and be a chance to be with that parent and have quality time together, whilst the carer is invigorated by catching up with friends which aides the reduction of feelings of isolation and being out of touch with themselves and the world around them.Activites such as going to the cinema, window shopping or going for a walk are things many of us take for granted all the time ,we are able to do them when we please. Freedom of choice and spontaneity are prized possessions and are frequently denied to carers, the loss of these freedoms compound the feelings of grief and possibly anger.

The same is true again of our friends and neighbours, carers can often find as they become increasingly housebound that they have fewer if any visitors. Too often the only visitors are from the medical profession, social services or voluntary organisations. Generally these callers have responsibility for the person affected with a memory problem and silently inside the carer is screaming "What about me?" From what I have been told, it appears that friends gradually withdraw from the lives of others due to their own ill health or more commonly, they just don't know what to say or do. They feel powerless; as none of us enjoy this feeling the temptation is to avoid it. We are human. Another reason could be the fear of being asked to do something, for example to sit with the person with a memory problem. They believe they would not know what to say and through the lack of knowledge of the condition are scared of "something happening". Few of us chose to readily take ourselves outside of our comfort zones. We like to feel that we are in control. To remedy this you might like to consider inviting friends you have not seen for a while for a coffee and catch-up. For the invitation to be accepted it would be useful if you told them that you missed their company and would enjoy a chinwag. I do mean a chinwag about all and sundry, not a whinge. We all avoid the moaners and the martyrs!

So close your eyes for a few moments and consider the help offered to you in the past that you were grateful to have. What was it about the help that you appreciated?

Was it when a rough and ready looking youth opened a door for you because you were laden with shopping? Or maybe you needed a lift somewhere and by chance conversation in the street or shop a neighbour offered unexpectedly to take you?

Listed below is a list of elements that allow help to be accepted;

- You are given choices.
- You feel that you have been listened to because what is offered is what is needed.
- The timing is spot on.
- There are no strings attached, or the conditions are acceptable to you.
- You feel the person understands your needs at that time.
- You feel a sense of reduced stress.
- The person is not being intrusive.
- The arrangements are mutually convenient.
- Both sides are clear to the commitment being made and the frequency.
- An honest exchange by both sides of what they want to get out of it.
- The giver of the help says if what is being done is O.K with them.
- The recipient is honest about what is needed.
- Clarity between NEED and desirable.(i.e. declaring you need to shop and collect a prescription versus It would be nice if I could window shop, or play bowls for a couple of hours)
- Collaboration is the key word NOT compromise.

When we think about people who have helped us the words we use to describe their efforts often include; kindness, generous, thoughtful, feel better, caring, happy, unconditional and benefitted from.

So close your eyes again and think about when help offered to you has not gone well. What was it about that help that was unacceptable? Did it make you feel inadequate? Or maybe you felt that the person was taking over.

Listed below is a list of elements that lead to the barriers whereby we reject help;

- The person is taking over things you are able to do.
- You are left feeling that you have an impossible debt to pay.
- The person has a tendency to let you down at the last moment.
- The time is restrictive and you feel it's not worth bothering.
- They burden you with their troubles.
- They don't do it your way.
- There are strings attached which you don't know how to get out of.
- You are made to feel inadequate.
- You feel guilty.

When we think about people whose help we have rejected and vowed never again, the words that come to mind are,useless,guilty,lazy,burden,sad,belittled,cruel,tension,difficult,friction,unhappy or bossy.

Giving and receiving help like I said earlier is full of pitfalls, but we can, if we take a few moments to stop and think about what it is we really want, we can begin to reduce negative experiences and embrace more positive ones.

When considering what help we are willing to accept we need to carefully think about who is best placed to satisfy the need. Pride may well have its place in our character but not at the expense of our health and overall wellbeing. We need to overcome any embarrassment and acknowledge which tasks we can hand over to someone else. Sometimes an outsider from the family is the best person because they are not emotionally involved. We need to be honest with ourselves first and then with others in what our expectations are, and declare if either the cost in money or emotion is too high a price to pay today. It is helpful if you feel the need to turn down an offer of help to leave the doors open for that person to come back, by saying, " thank you for your kind offer, but not at the moment thank you, but who knows maybe another time would be nice" this way no one is rejected or loses face.

Up until this point the focus of acceptable help has been centred on the carer. What about the person with a memory problem? So often I come across situations where this person somehow slips into being no longer verbally considered. This is not a deliberate act of cruelty on anyone's part, more where self preservation of the carer leads to the scales becoming unbalanced.

It is no surprise really that this state occurs. If a couple have been married for thirty plus years there is a lot of familiarity in place. Both know the daily routine and moods of the other, each others likes and dislikes and patterns of behaviour and conversation are well established. So why does a problem arise? The answer lies in the nature of memory problems. The carer becomes the decision maker, what to eat, when to eat it, the list goes on and increases with the passage of the condition. As the person with a memory problem is stripped of their reasoning skills and the ability to learn new information it becomes increasingly difficult for daily "normal" conversation to take place. In fact it can became quite monosyllabic and be no more than a series of questions and answers. As the carer is "in the know" they find themselves reducing the level of communication, so the skills that the person still has access to may become rusty and lost through lack of use, compounded by the progression of the condition. A double whammy so to speak. It may sound false to talk to yourself out loud but you can still talk to the person. It is tiring and I guess can be likened to hospital visiting which often feels strenuous and stilted but there is no reason not to mentally stimulate the person and share with them some of your thoughts and observations, in particular daily chit chat. I totally accept that carers can reach a point when they can no long share their fears and worries with the person as this leads to distress all round. This is why you both need breaks, some fresh stimulating conversation, to energise you both and as a result have more to share.

Carers have frequently told me that they cannot have a break because they feel guilty about having a nice time without the person. What I say to them is "how do you know that the person won't enjoy the break?" The person with a memory problem generally does not stop having feelings. They lose the ability to express them, particularly in words. Communication is also about using all our senses. Sometimes their behaviour is a reflection of the frustrations they have due to the condition, or the way they feel that they are treated. At the end of the day all behaviour is a form of communication. Instead of feeling that you are having a break because you need it, why not turn it on its head and tell the person that you are giving them a break and change of company and/or scenery. Meeting their needs as well as your own can be very rewarding for both of you. By trying this you can both bask in positive help and all those nice feel good words mentioned earlier.

Go on give it a go......... and enjoy.

PROBLEMS...WE ALL HAVE THEM!

Problem from Greek... *problemat,*
"projection, obstacle" literally
"thing thrown in front"

So what is a problem other than than a time consuming nuisance? A problem is when you are faced with a set of circumstances that you do not know how to satisfactorily resolve. What is a problem for one person might well be a total non issue for another. The reason we find caring situations apparently beyond dealing with is often due to two things, firstly we do not have the necessary information and secondly the human nature that is, a tendency to protect others we care about, by second guessing their views. This strategy can lead to all sorts of complications. This leads to the question "what can be done?" The first thing is to decide just how important it is to do anything. If it is a matter of someone's safety or health then either the emergency services or your doctor or social services have to be the first point of contact. It is a good idea to have a list of essential phone numbers to hand. If ever you are concerned please do not hesitate to seek advice, and do so promptly so as to prevent a minor treatable concern becoming more complicated. Generally most people know how to handle critical situations, but then there is every thing else that life throws at you, these are never so easy to manage and can lead to sleepless nights fraught with worry. Sadly worry does nothing to achieve the desired outcome and can lead to complications within the family or friendships as well as health conditions being aggravated. In the small wee hours of the night the object of our concern grows beyond any manageable size and as we are talking to ourselves we go round and round in circles leading in the morning to tiredness and exasperation. The more tired we become the less able we can see the wood for the trees.

On most occasions the solution is usually best found within the person who is experiencing difficulties. This is because it is that person who has to handle the situation, and the outcome. It is no good being bombarded by well meaning people telling you what to do, but it is useful to listen with an open mind to their suggestions as the principle of their idea may have some useful components that you can personalise. It's a good idea to sleep on it and consider your options with their contributions in mind. It could provide the foundations to dealing with your problem. This approach allows you to look at ways you may not have otherwise considered and allows the person to feel that they have been of service to you. A win –win situation. At the end of the day only you know what is acceptable to you and what you believe is unmanageable. There is often not a right or wrong more usually it is a case of "I can live with that" or "there is no way that is O.K for me". In the attempt to preserve relationships it is also wise to avoid saying things such as "It's alright for you, you don't have to..."Despite being engulfed by your problem you need to try to remember that we all have different levels of tolerance, ability, knowledge and experience to draw on, it is not as straight for ward as one person being right and therefore the other person is wrong.

One method of resolving difficult issues is to get a piece of paper and write down all the things you could do and then consider the pros and cons to each one. For example you might be wondering what to do about having a disturbed night sleep..........

So..... on a piece of paper you might write;

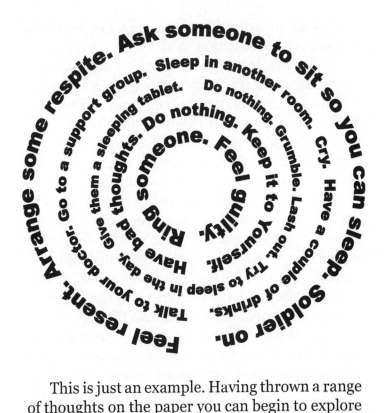

Arrange some respite. Ask someone to sit so you can sleep. Soldier on. Feel resent. Go to a support group. Sleep in another room. Cry. Have a couple of drinks. Talk to your doctor. Give them a sleeping tablet. Do nothing. Grumble. Lash out. Try to sleep in the day. Have bad thoughts. Do nothing. Keep it to yourself. Ring someone. Feel guilty.

This is just an example. Having thrown a range of thoughts on the paper you can begin to explore the consequences of each option. At the end of the day or thought process the piece of incriminating paper can be destroyed....hopefully you will not be destroyed but feel stronger and more positive. Doing nothing is an option but could come with a surprise price tag. By doing nothing you could be writing a cheque that you health cannot afford to pay. The result being your worst nightmare, for example you may be at this point dead set against the thought of "putting" the person into respite for a week whilst you top up your batteries, for fear of having betrayed them. The danger is that if you do not take the opportunity to recharge your battery's a short term disruption to daily life could spiral out of control, leading to the long term possibility of permanent care, becoming the only solution. Should your health become compromised and you fall ill the very thing that you wish to avoid could potentially become a reality. The cruel and harsh truth is that you cannot continue to care 24/7 for your loved one if you are six foot under.

Part of the process of solving a problem is to know your bottom line. Knowing your self with honesty and being clear about what is no longer acceptable whilst realising there may be more than one option and there has to be some give and take. So that takes us back a moment to the previous pages about help, allow yourself time to reflect on what works for you and yours, remembering to not discount untried options. Once you have identified possible options to explore from your pros and cons list, it may emerge that you have a clearer idea about what to do next. Circle on your list the unacceptable and put a smiling face by the options to be actioned. Now think who or what might be most useful. Don't worry there may well be more questions than obvious answers at this point. Talking to someone who is not emotionally involved very often helps to give clarity and not uncommonly the process of telling a stranger the issues that perplex you, is not only therapeutic but also is half the work done. The very process of hearing yourself saying out loud what the issues are will in itself shed light as how to move forward.

This can lead to greater clarity of perspective with regard to your current levels of tolerance and ability to cope.

The next stage is to contemplate the triggers of your problem. Still using the example of having a disturbed nights sleep, is it because the person you care for has a prostrate problem and they wake in the night to use the toilet and then think it is time to get up having temporarily recharged their batteries? Or maybe they have catnapped through the day? (Possibly due to boredom) and therefore are unable to readily get back to sleep, or maybe the interaction between the two of you on waking stimulates them and disrupts the ability to resettle for the night. It could be a combination of all of the above.

It could also be due to being too hot or not warm enough. They might be hungry or thirsty. Maybe the room is stuffy and needs ventilating. Our environment can be the cause of making us restless, which translates itself into difficult behaviour. All behaviour is a form of communication. It is possible that they are confused and disoriented upon waking, knowing they need the toilet but not recognising where they are, so having used the toilet are still unsettled by the environment that seems at that moment in time alien to them ,hence causing reluctance to go back to sleep. We have all experienced those few moments when we stay somewhere unfamiliar, when it takes a while to get our bearings and this is a common experience for people with a memory problem, especially just after waking up.

In the process of resolving problems it is negative to use blame. Blame means that there is fault. It is not their fault that they are disturbing your sleep. I know it may feel as though they are being deliberately stubborn and awkward, in fact they are trying to tell you something. The night is not the time for a discussion on the problem. The night is for minimal disruption and a cuddle to reassure.

In this scenario it might be an option to talk to your doctor and have some night medication to give the person to enhance sleep. I would suggest that in discussion with your G.P, it is not given at 9.30pm when they go to bed, but midnight or so when the first go to the toilet. Given with a small cup of warm milk (taken with you to bed in a flask) and a cuddle of reassurance can be most effective for both of you. The following six to seven hours of sleep helping both of you face the next day in better rested condition. I would also look to ways of reducing the number of catnaps in a day and ensuring enough physical activity. It is vital that you speak with your G.P about the disrupted night routine and how best to manage any medication. Medication is something that should not be juggled without medical advice.

Women not uncommonly talk to friends and family, but for our older generation of men they find themselves at a loss, having been raised by the Victorian attitude that men do not talk about emotions and certainly not in public. Often referred to as the typically British quirk of a "stiff upper lip". This can lead to older men who are carers for someone with a memory problem to become very isolated and distressed. How do they overcome the things that are a cause of concern? When the one person they could talk to is no longer able to engage in meaningful decision making. It can be most upsetting. Men may be from Mars and women from Venus but the common ground when it comes to the caring role is vast. It can feel incredibly disloyal talking about your loved one's short comings within their ear shot hence the need to be able to talk if you wish away from their hearing. Even though women may be renowned for being able to talk!!!! I have often heard tales of woe from women who have found themselves socially isolated as friends and neighbours no longer call or pass the time of day. The reason being that those friends and neighbours just do not know what to say. In our society we often pass a neighbour calling out "hello, how are you?" often not stopping to hear the answer in case we become entrenched in the ongoing complaints of the women who lives two doors down and always moans. Does that sound familiar? Which are you the moaner or the person making the excuse? Saying "I can't stop, must catch up soon" knowing full well that you have no intention of doing so, and as soon as you get home saying to your loved one, "You'll never guess who I saw today dear"? And launch into how you evaded stopping for a twenty minute chat. Saying "You know what she's like". Often people do not mean to moan, it is that they have few occasions to be able to share the day to day ups and downs we all experience. We can all be guilty of taking these apparently small things for granted...that is until we are denied access to them. Remember there are no medals for a martyr. By spending a few moments listening to the person and showing genuine warmth you could walk away with your halo a little brighter in the knowledge that you have made someone's day a bit more bearable. If you are the moaner then an option available is to invite the person in for a chat to see your garden or have a cuppa, and be upfront by saying how much you miss day to day chats.

Whether you are a male or female carer you belong to the human race which in the main is a social beast who grows in the company of others. Something to consider is joining a social group, here again you have two options, firstly a group for carers in a similar position as yourself, or secondly joining something which is of interest to you and get totally away from what is going on at home. For the second scenario the options are endless, limited only by how brave you to give it a go. The first option is one that some people are wary of, maybe you falsely believe you will be made to say something against you will. This is not the case. Support Groups run by the Alzheimer's Society are run by competent and compassionate people who have a genuine understanding. It is important to know that the Alzheimer's Society is available to both carers and the cared for any memory problem not just those affected by Alzheimer's disease. You do not need a diagnosis to receive support or access information from them. What is more important are the people who attend, as they truly appreciate what it is like caring for someone with a memory problem 24/7. This is the place where there is safety in numbers, where you are not judged and you do not have to justify yourself. You also get the chance to make new acquaintances and have a laugh....which as we all know(after a good cup of tea) is the best medicine.

REMEMBER REMEMBER

Remember, remember the fifth of November
Gunpowder, treason and plot..........

For any thing to be remembered it has to have been learnt in the first place. If we consider the brain as a storage container for information then it has to have been filed first before it can be retrieved. I think of it like this, a book is a storage container of data in a code, we need to understand that code, by that I mean comprehend the written word before we can interpret the content of that book. So if the book is written in Spanish and you do not understand Spanish you will not be able to decode the content of that book. Whereas if that book is written in your language you are better equipped in interpreting the code it contains. If there are words that you do not know the meaning of then you might ask someone, use a dictionary or make your own interpretation so it makes sense to you based on prior knowledge and experience.

So learning is the process of putting the information into storage and memory (or remembering) is the process of retrieving the information.

People with a memory problem have difficulty

in the three main areas of memory which include the storing, the holding onto and the retrieving what has been put into storage. The access code is denied to them. By the same token if the information has never been put into storage then it is not there to be retrieved.

The learnt information for people with a memory problem is stored but the pathway to being able to retrieve it is damaged and therefore only some elements may be recalled to mind, making conversation appear fragmented and nonsensical to the listener.

If we imagine the old fashioned telephonist at a switchboard for a moment...................... You ask a person a question which is like dialling a telephone number, the telephonist answers "hold on a moment while I try to connect you". The person you are calling is the information you are trying to access, but unfortunately their lines are down and therefore they are unable to retrieve the required information and offer it to you.

For people with a memory problem in decoding a situation, or something that is expected of them as well as conversation they often rely on prior knowledge and experience of yesteryear to explain today's conundrums. This may be very funny as it may be jumbled to the observer but it might be very frustrating for the person as they do not realise the source of hilarity. They may become sensitive or even hostile if they feel that they are being laughed at, as do we all.

If we consider memory as either a short term

or long term storage agreement then the complex nature of forgetting is a little easier to explain. It is possible that as the information was only in temporary storage (by this we mean that recall is only available for up to a minute without rehearing the information) and if it was not transferred to long term storage then as a result it has been lost. It could be that it was transferred to longer term storage but no record of the route it took has been kept so it takes a lot of searching to locate it and there are many other interesting snippets that look similar on the way which distracts the search. It is possible that obstacles either on the route to finding the lost information or on the journey back adds to the confusion. Finally it may be that the memory fades away so that it is no longer available. The temporary storage is what you will often hear as short term memory. An example of this might be asking the person what they had for breakfast in the late morning, they reply "oh the usual dear," if you probe a little further becoming more persistent in wanting detail then the person may become defensive or tetchy. Their response was a clever use of self preservation aimed at fending off further questioning as their retrieval system has a failure. It is also a human nature response to protect ourselves from looking stupid in front of others.

The memory is very complex and there are a wide range of gadgets available that the person may find useful to help prompt them. One thing that tends to happen fairly early on is that the carer realises that the person forgets simple information and may struggle with easy instructions. How each person is affected varies a lot. Writing on a message board or leaving notes as to what time you will be back can be very helpful and reassuring. Some people use fridge magnets to leave messages, the most important thing is whatever method you employ, is the message is left where it is likely to found. Try to consider the person's routine in your absence to determine the best place to leave the note. Ask them where they think might be best.

As you may have discovered the long term memory seems to be more in tact .This is because memories from the past were formed and stored before the damage took place. Indeed often repeated stories from years long gone are a firm favourite to the person with a memory problem. It is due to non corruption of early learnt data that is safely stored in the long term memory and that has regular use that someone can continue to safely drive a car but may not be able to change the T.V.channel with the remote control.

LET'S TAKE A WALK DOWN MEMORY LANE

What is this life, if full of care,
We have no time to stand and stare.

W.H Davies (1871-1940)

It might sound old fashioned to suggest making a scrapbook, but it is the principle that I am proposing to you and friends and family. Scrapbooks are one way of preserving memories, a bit like a jumbled diary, and that is the essence of this activity. The idea is to encourage family and friends to contribute to this unique treasure chest of memories that can be revisited time and again. As the person with a memory problem will blissfully recount stories from the past, and aided by prompts may be able to connect to occasions, some more recent, otherwise lost.

The scrapbook should contain nuggets of clues to a life gone by, and enable the person sharing the trip down memory lane to not have to start from scratch, instead having a handful of treasures to look over with the person. It is a way of enabling their memories to be captured and cherished over and again, helping to remain in touch with the real person locked away by memory loss. It goes some way to making the person valid not invalid.

There is no right or wrong way to achieve this scrapbook. Ideally though you should be aware of two main elements which are those that are the person's memories, and very differently those that are your memories.

Carers and relatives often find it very distressing when they clearly remember a significant event, lets say a grandchild's wedding, but to Granddad there is a void around the occasion. Typically various people present say "ohh go on Granddad you must remember when..." and poor Granddad becomes flustered and if possible removes himself from the conversation, or feigns sleep to avoid further probing. Granddad is not trying to hurt your feelings but, his emotions at the time were not as overwhelming as yours. It brings a whole new meaning to lost in translation! You can close you eyes and cast your minds eye over a range of various events of the occasion.... but if you speak to others present they may remember some of what you do but also things that passed you by. Why is this? Well ask yourself what are the dominant emotions around any given memory? I suspect it will be one of a few basic emotions of happiness, fear, anxiety, guilt, laughter, sadness, jealousy or embarrassment. If Granddad had a less definite emotion to the event then it is harder for him to recollect. So, back to the scrapbook, you may find pictures help to prompt a connection, as might music, especially if it had been familiar to them; this is to aid the sensory memory. In today's world technology is moving at a fast pace and we now have digital photograph frames which are a wonderful way of storing magical moments, just remember to include their moments not only yours.

Things that can enhance memory recollection should include all five senses of sight, hearing, touch taste and smell. A scrapbook will only provoke the sense of sight by the use of the written word or pictures. Examples of this are photographs and poetry. Recently a lot of research has been done around how powerful music is to stimulate memories. For the generation who World War Two hold mixed memories a C.D of wartime melodies may access hidden stories long stored away, a word of caution though as it may unleash floods of tears too. This need not be a bad thing as long as those present can cope with, and have time for an emotional episode. To activate the sense of taste treating the person to meals that were firm favourites such as boiled beef and carrots with dumplings or jam roly poly and custard can be a way of generating conversation and memories. To promote memories using touch creating a shoe box filled with an assortment of things from pine cones, sea shells, old buttons, old coins or memorabilia from the trade that person was in can help pass many a happy hour for all involved and give insight into someone's life. Let's say it is a woman who has a memory problem, things like old kitchen implements in a magazine, or pieces of different textured material remnants along with buttons and reels of cotton or maybe knitting needles or a crochet hook with old patterns enable conversation of days gone by. These objects are in keeping with her role in her generation, not yours as a modern 21st century person.

Also visits to rural museums which often have tea rooms can be a pleasurable way to pass a couple of hours. On these outings if allowed by the venue taking a photo of the person and you there can be added to the scrapbook. (Include yourselves in a photo to help place you both in the togetherness of the memory)

If you do not fancy a scrapbook you might like to consider compiling a family favourite recipe book. Do include the how to do and the timings. If it is Mum or Nan who has a memory problem you might be able to sell the idea to them by expressing a desire to learn the family favourite dishes. In time if Dad or Granddad need to become chief cook and bottle washer they could be very grateful to have inside information.

Another excellent reason for creating a scrapbook, or shoebox of items or a C.D is that should the loved one come to need to moved into permanent care it helps the staff get to know the person more easily, as the do not have to ask direct probing questions but can sit with them and look together at the treasure chest of goodies, in turn giving the person some validity and respect which would lead to an increased quality of life.

It helps to make care personal.

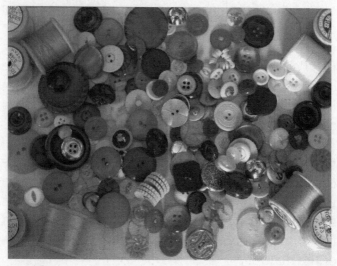

What I am about to suggest may initially sound provocative to you especially if you are in the early stages of your caring journey. I make the suggestion to hopefully bring you some comfort and solace in times to come. If you are further into your journey it is still not too late. What I propose is that you the carer make a scrapbook or album for yourself of good times, your hopes and dreams. The little things that make you smile or capture the essence of your special relationship with the person you are caring for. The dementias are a cruel unforgiving set of conditions that day by day slowly rob you both of a life once planned. By creating your own treasure chest of magical moments you can, in times of loss once again touch the real person. On days were you have been driven to despair when your loved one asks for the twentieth time in an hour the same question

and you are besieged by unthinkable thoughts......
reach for the recording of their laughter, or photo
of happier times and reconnect to the real person,
who is cruelly lost to you due to the ever marching
onwards of their dementia.

So just to be clear two collections have been
suggested, one for you the carer to enable you to
hold dear all that is special about your relationship
to the person with a memory problem, the second
for the person with a memory problem to help
others understand the uniqueness and individual
aspects of the person should there come a time that
they are no longer able to represent themselves.

If you make a DVD or C.D of the person please
remember that there are laws and they can only
be used for personal use, as the person has to give
their permission for this and have the capacity
to consent to it being viewed publically. In other
words it is for private viewing/listening only.

There is a popular saying at the moment
which is ....use it before you lose it. The brain
and its functions are complex but it is a part of
the body that we tend to disregard as needing to
be exercised. Not only are a healthy diet, fresh
air and physical exercise essential for a healthy
mind but so is mental exercise. There are several
things that could be done. Jigsaws are good for
visualising space and shapes. Games such as
dominoes and cards are good for promoting
memory and sequencing and planning. I-spy,
hangman crosswords, Sudoku are all positive
ways of stimulating the grey cells. If preferred you

could do rounds of naming animals or flowers for each letter of the alphabet. If there are a few of you then Grandmas Basket is good fun for all ages and not just at Christmas. Nursery rhymes also take us back to not only our childhood but those of our children too. Word association games are not only amusing but good exercise. In essence what were popularly known as parlour games, still hold great value today. With this type of amusement you are limited only by the boundaries of your speed of memory recollection and your imagination. Try to be patient with each player as they search their memory banks, this is not meant as speed trials.

Carers and visitors often forget to allow themselves to have fun too; it is as though the task of conversing is seen as a laborious task to be carried out. It is a way of reducing the daily stresses, it should be valued and cherished , by slowing down and allowing yourselves to not consider it a waste of time and feel you should be doing something else, you can positively enhance everyone's wellbeing. Conversation has immeasurable benefits...add some laughter and you are well on the way to having the recipe for a pleasurable few hours. Time will fly.

THE LOST ART OF CONVERSATION

I think that generosity is the essence of friendship.
From The Devoted Friend by Oscar Wilde.

When we find ourselves in the position of sitting or visiting a person with the memory problem conversation can feel false and stilted. Once we have taken a few moments to ask how they are today and in true British fashion discuss the weather. What comes next? Oh yes a quick telling of a recent family activity or Mrs Brown down the road going into hospital with ingrown toenails....but that's only taken ten minutes. Maybe a few lines on how the grass needs cutting and accepting a cup of tea and biscuits. Already you are clock watching and frantically trying to think of some reason to cut this visit short. It is time to stop being so busy and do one thing at a time and enjoy it for what it is. Multitasking is not always clever when it is at the expense of not really paying heed to the job in hand. Talking and sharing and listening skills are fast becoming a dying breed in today's world of go go go.

Time to close your eyes again, for a few moments and let yourself drift, thinking back to times gone by. Consider magical moments and remember smells and sights and sounds from the past. What wonders did you touch that linger in the dusty corners of your memory? We all have hordes of nostalgic collections, no matter whether we are 12 or 92. Join in with the person in reliving their memories, below are clusters of objects and products and well known names from the past.

Entertainment..

The Odeon cinema.
Sing Something Simple.   Russ Conway and a five fingered vamp.
Mrs Mills.   Victor Sylvester.
The Tiller Girls.
Sunday Night at the London Palladium.   Black and white T.V.
B.B.C. World Service.   Mrs Dale's Diary.
Over The Garden Wall.

The Kitchen...

Spam.   Horlicks.   Ovaltine.   Stones Ginger Wine.   Typhoo Tea.
Colman's mustard powder.   Powdered Eggs.
Buying butter in ½ lb wraps.   Scotts Porridge.
Marmite.   Camp Coffee.   No bananas.   No Oranges. Oxo.   Persil or Omo washing powder.
Dolly Blue. Robin's Starch.

Bassets Liquorice Allsorts. Sharps toffees. Corona lemonade. Tate and Lyle golden syrup as well as sugar. Brasso. Bread and dripping.

In The Home..

Jeyes Fluid. Andrew's Liver Salts. Epsom salts. Cherry Blossom shoe polish. Spills to light the cooker. Gas hair tong. Woman's Own Magazine. Peoples Friend Magazine.. Patience Strong poems . Cotton Handkerchiefs. Gravy browning to create stocking lines. Parma Violets. Having a larder. Outside toilet. Izal toilet paper. Dr Whites Sanitary towels. Pond's cold cream. T.C.P. Pears soap. Flat iron. Singer sewing machines.Sylko threads. Thimbles for sewing. Darning socks. Atco lawnmowers.

Lifestyle..

4711 eau de cologne. Chanel No5. Old Spice. Lady's wore gloves and had handbags. Sunday best. Market day. Wash day. Bake day. Makeson. Brylcreme. Wet shave. N.H.S. Dog racing. Dark floors. The Parlour. Carriage prams. Hornby train sets. Wearing an apron. Scrubbing the front door step. Coal fires. At the dentist having gas via a red rubber mask. Grow your own veg. Lyons Coffee house. Homemade rugs. Midwives did home deliveries. Terry nappies. Home deliveries of fish, eggs, coal, groceries, bread and milk in glass milk bottles. Zippo lighters. Watches that had to be wound each day. Lino flooring. Walk ,cycle or take the bus ,tram or train. Steam trains.diddly dee diddly dum. Meccano.Woodbine, Senior Service, Players cigarettes. Collecting cigarette cards. Clark shoes. Prudential. Ford cars. Esso.Shell. Dunlop tyres. Kodak Brownie camera. Sutton seeds. Vinyl records. H.M.V.Fish and Chips in newspaper. £.s.d. lbs and oz. times tables to 12. Inches. Lb bag of nails. Yard of sand. Telegrams. Postal Orders. Pigeon racing. Silver screen stars. Silver sixpence. Threepenny bit. Going to bed wearing a hair net. Gay meant happy.

The World at Large...

Air raid shelters. Blackout. Sirens. Blitz. Edward and Mrs Simpson. Churchill. Kitchener..your country needs you. Gas masks. Titanic.
The Maginot Line. The Siegfried Line. Charles Lindbergh's Spirit of St Louis. Alexander Fleming's discovery of Penecillin.Noel Coward. Walt Disney's Mickey Mouse.Ghandi.Vietnam.

The lists are by no means complete but here to help you get going. There might be things written in the lists that have no meaning for you what so ever, perhaps you could begin by introducing one or two that are vaguely familiar to you and discover a whole new world, but more importantly discover the rich memories of the person with a memory problem. Not forgetting those memories of not just sights and sounds but also smells and the feel of things. Many fabrics were coarse and itchy due to the wool content and manufacturing process as well as washing techniques.

The next collection is put together from a different angle for you to use. It is an assortment of things that are now readily available and often taken for granted but were alien 50 years ago. The world we live in is developing so fast, the technology is phenomenal and pressing forward at an alarming rate. It is impossible for the person with a memory problem to take a lot of the new world on board, as a feature of their condition is not only poor concentration but a reduced ability to learn new things. They find safety and comfort in their past where life moved at a much slower pace and everyone was doing the same and owned very similar possessions as choice was more restricted. So in no particular order.........here goes..........

TV's with remote control. Mobile phones. Microwave. Dishwasher. Satellite Television. Cruising holidays. Holidays abroad. T-bags. Pizza. McDonalds. Disney World. Pasta. Sushi. David Attenbrough.ISA's Home computers. Hover mowers. Power showers. Digital photo frames. Concorde. Plastic surgery. Punk rock. Moon landings. Body piercings. Botox. Nelson Mandela. The Berlin wall coming down. Euro. Channel tunnel. Chewing gum. School targets.En-suite bathrooms. Contact lenses. Margaret Thatcher. Tumble dryers. Ikea.Jacuzzi.Reality T.V shows.

So now you have a wide range of topics to explore. There is a lot of talking to be done. To truly have a rewarding conversation we need to ensure that we also do some listening. Before we can really listen we need to settle down to the job at hand.

CAUTION; Beware the modern day curse of multi-tasking. Women in today's fast pace of life find themselves excelling at doing more than one job at a time. Or are they? It can leave you feeling dissatisfied as too much is going on at once. We forget to allow the answer phone to pick up the message, we answer in case it is important. We moan about the difficulties of juggling a big "must do immediately" work load that can't wait. Stop for a moment, catch your breath, put some fuel back into the tank and allow yourself to do one thing at a time and enjoy it.Multi-tasking can be very damaging to the art of meaningful conversation and companionship. This is because we do not give real value to the here and now.Multi-tasking means that your attention is not with what you are currently doing but several steps ahead of the game. Being what appears to one step ahead of the game is often not really valuing to what or who we are tending to.Multi-tasking can be a bit like turning a hot tap on too much to wash-up and being scalded by hot greasy water. Ouch. If we are multi-tasking we are distracted from what is really being said or done. Here, now, this minute.

A definition of, "to listen" is to make a conscious effort to hear and to concentrate on what someone is saying. Again in today's fast pace of life people do not listen as well as they would like to think they do. Really listening is tiring. To understand speech we use our sense of sight just as much as our ears to hear. We watch the speaker's mouth move. If we are denied this second visual aid we can often mishear what has actually been said. For people who have a hearing deficit or poor vision this can make conversation more difficult. If there is a lot of back round noise this also reduces the clarity of our hearing. So large family gatherings can become an ordeal for those affected by visual or hearing problems, and if you couple this with a memory problem where the ability to concentrate and process information is damaged, it becomes easier to understand why someone may be reluctant to be in that environment. Just try for a moment standing back to back with someone and hold a conversation.....it is very difficult.(if you do try this exercise please do not talk about anything important because ,as you will both discover it is very hard to concentrate when you are deprived of all senses.)

There are other barriers to us being able to chat. We tend to believe that everyday conversation goes like this;

I speak and you listen.   Then I listen while you speak.   In reality what happens is; I speak, while you listen, you plan your response, you get distracted, you day dream, you review your original planned answer, and when I stop you reply. There is a lot going on. So if someone has a memory problem and is distracted or does not get the chance to answer when the thought that is in their head materialises then the two- way conversation falls apart. For the person to be able to interact verbally they need time to be able to access their response without being pressured by too many prompts which distracts their processes. This applies in particular to someone with Alzheimer's disease whereas someone who has had a stroke may be able to access the thought more easily but struggle to vocalise it due to having to relearn how to talk (depending on which area of the brain was affected).Both conditions have their frustrations, for speaker's and listeners.

Another clue as to what a person has to say is their body language. Think about the number of times you have heard someone say something but been left feeling confused. Mixed message often occur when people say one thing but their body language tells us something else. They say our eyes are the windows to our soul. You may have noticed a slight rise in an eyebrow, or a twinkle of the eye which allows a subtext to take place. Subtle facial expressions are interpreted from a very early age and we rely on our understanding of this language to help us decode the spoken word. The lack of patience for example is noticeable, not only facially, but maybe emphasised with finger tapping or knee twitching to name but two. Or maybe their eyes look sad and teary, but when asked how they are the reply is "I'm fine". When we think about people we know, it is the subtle little expressions and actions that give us a clue to how they are feeling. People with a memory problem often continue to give us these clues as long as we do not stop noticing them. More can be expressed with an action or reaction than words. We need to fine tune our patience in allowing people time to express themselves. We need to allow them to use it all the while they can.

It is also essential to not underestimate what someone with a dementia understands. If you need to make an observation with another family member it is best to do it out of earshot. Sensitivity is required so as not to make the person paranoid. None of us like being talked about, especially if we believe it to be derogatory.

SILENCE IS GOLDEN

"Silence is golden but my eyes still see."
From the song by The Tremeloes.

Other than being the song title to a well know song what does silence mean to you? Are you someone who likes noise around most of the time? Or do you enjoy periods of quiet so you can explore your thoughts or pleasantly daydream? Silence is an essential part of conversation. People with a memory problem need quiet moments within a conversation to retrieve their thoughts, or experience the memory that has been reactivated.

Silences are important to reduce the number of obstacles we inadvertently lay in the path of someone trying to find the buried information. It is a bit like being in overload. Too much external interference prevents us remembering. This is something we all experience at times when we have too much on our plate. Many of us have gone upstairs planning to do something and then stopped. If we retrace our steps the intended job comes back to mind. People with a memory problem need uninterrupted time to retrieve information.

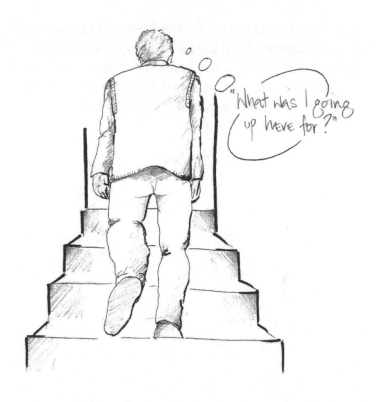

It could be more productive to re-prompt as to where you were in the conversation, i.e. "Granddad we were just talking about....."And offering him the chance to re-enter the chat with minimal distractions.

Why not allow yourself some time to reflect on the usual way that you converse with the person with a memory problem .Consider if sometimes there could be a more enjoyable and caring way in which it could take place. Please do not be harsh on yourself if these few chapters have helped you see another way of doing things. All learning is positive. You can only do the best you can at any given moment in time. This means taking into account how well and rested you are. You are important, you are on, what is possibly a sharp learning curve, your needs are paramount too.

RESPITE IS NOT A DIRTY WORD

Respite means a brief interval of rest for recovery

I suspect that if I have the audacity to suggest to you that you need some respite that you might be tempted to snap this book shut. Please don't.

For all of us to maintain our well-being and a reasonable contentment with our lot; we need several things

- We need Air, Water, and Food.

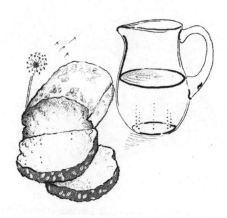

- We need a roof over our heads, a place where we feel safe and secure.

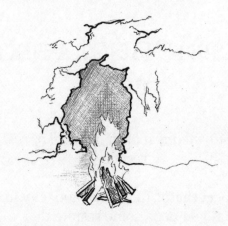

- We need adequate quality sleep.

- We need to feel loved; this ranges from cuddles to a satisfying sex life.

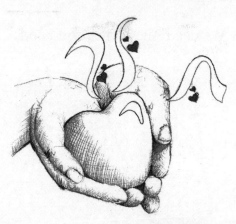

- We need to have a sense of belonging not

only to our family but to our community. We like to fit in and be accepted.

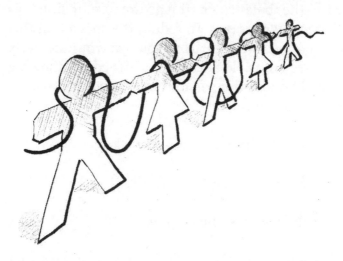

- Collectively this helps to build our self esteem and resourcefulness.

- When we have all of the above, it enables us to gain a sense of value and give a meaning to our lives. It promotes a vitality and playfulness in our demeanour. It makes us feel connected to our place in the world.

It makes us human.
(*This is known as Maslow's hierarchy of needs, A.H. Maslow was an American psychologist. 1908-1970*)

Taking the above into account it becomes

easier to understand points in our lives whereby we become dissatisfied. When we become unhappy with the balance of things we are defined as "being out of sorts". To reduce the speed that this can happen in the caring role we can take early positive steps. This can be achieved by allowing ourselves and the person being cared for to keep the equilibrium.

We do this by having a break.

By recharging our batteries.

By having some respite.

I am not suggesting in these early days that formal care homes are what are needed. But I do suggest that as this is probably what you do

not want, so steps need to be taken in reducing a breakdown in the carer/cared for situation.

The way in which we structure the day can allow both parties to keep their sense of being alive, which validates their existence.

Much better than being made to feel worthless and devalued.

We considered in the chapter "The Caring Role" that when you were part of the workforce that you had a job description and annual leave. Now you are a member of a different workforce, a silent band of devoted workers who operate behind closed doors. In effect your loved one is your employer. They need you to operate efficiently. To do this for the unknown duration you need to look after yourself. By doing this, you are better placed to maintain your role as a carer.

You as the carer are in many ways the most important person in the equation. If you fall ill or struggle to cope then what you do not want to happen (i.e. the person having to be placed in a care home) is unfortunately exactly what might happen. No one knows how they will cope until faced with the situation. We can however enhance our own well-being by allowing ourselves time out. This does not make you a bad or weak person. It means that you are human. To maintain a complete person as we saw at the beginning of this chapter you need all the listed elements, in balance, in your life.

We would not ask a plumber to do an electrician's job. Therefore why do we expect ourselves to be natural knowledgeable carers? It is not realistic. All common sense can be thrown out of the window when we are emotionally involved.

It can also be surprisingly challenging if you have prior knowledge of caring as it can lull you into a false sense of expectation as to how things will pan out. Life is never that straight forward. As each individual has their own life experiences and health history, it leads to all caring journey's being unique. Granted there will be common threads. For certain it will throw up new unexpected challenges. Your relationship with each person varies, the emotional attachment varies, which produces mixed emotions.

Let's look at way in which you can recharge your batteries....

Employ your subconscious....because your subconscious specialises in finding solutions to your problems. So place your faith in it, and give your conscious mind a rest. In other words we can think about a problem too much. If you have worries, distract yourself and let your mind sort things out it's self.

∞∞∞∞∞∞∞∞∞∞∞∞∞∞∞∞∞∞∞∞∞∞∞∞∞∞∞∞∞∞∞∞∞∞∞∞

Press the roof of your mouth with your tongue for the count of 10 to release tension. Tense people have tense jaw muscles so by doing this exercise through the day helps relieve some tension.

∞∞∞∞∞∞∞∞∞∞∞∞∞∞∞∞∞∞∞∞∞∞∞∞∞∞∞∞∞∞

Visit your local churches and absorb the peace.

∞∞∞∞∞∞∞∞∞∞∞∞∞∞∞∞∞∞∞∞∞∞∞∞∞∞∞∞∞

Shed a few tears....crying gives relief to built up tension and releases toxins that build up when we are stressed. For all of you gentlemen I realise this may go against the grain of your upbringing but it will do you good.

∞∞∞∞∞∞∞∞∞∞∞∞∞∞∞∞∞∞∞∞∞∞∞∞∞∞∞∞

Take pleasure in life's simple delights. They are free. The dew on the morning grass.

The smell of new cut lawns. Blossom on the trees. Have a bird table. Sunsets, especially red ones bode well, as they bring the promise of good weather the next day.

∞∞∞∞∞∞∞∞∞∞∞∞∞∞∞∞∞∞∞∞∞∞∞∞∞

A cup of warm water will calm you and re-hydrate you almost immediately which will give you a sense of wellbeing, as well as improving thinking and decision making tasks.

∞∞∞∞∞∞∞∞∞∞∞∞∞∞∞∞∞∞∞∞∞∞∞∞∞

Smile.....even strangers will smile back. It not only gives you a warm glow inside but eases tension. It takes less facial muscles to smile than frown.

∞∞∞∞∞∞∞∞∞∞∞∞∞∞∞∞∞∞∞∞∞∞∞∞

Morning cups..........when getting up each morning, say out loud several times "my cup is half full" and plan how you might top it up. May your cup runneth over and never run dry.

THE DEMENTIA UMBERELLA

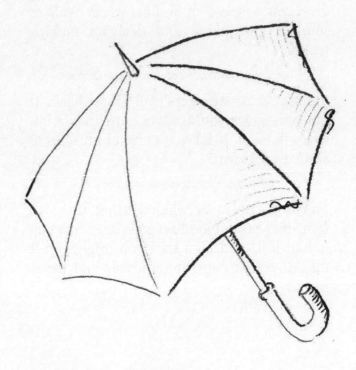

Time for the science bit. To me it is important in simple terms to be clear about what dementia is. Dementia is not a normal part of aging, although it is more common in older people it does not happen because you are old. In a nutshell dementia is a progressive decline in cognitive functioning caused by disease of the brain or damage to the brain. O.K I hear you say "cognitive functioning" can I have that in English please?

Cognitive functioning includes;

- How we use language,
- Our ability to concentrate,
- How we plan ,arrange and organise ourselves,
- Our use of memory in learning it, storing it and recalling it.
- Our ability to recognise where we are, or what time of day or year it is.
- Our ability to accurately judge the space we live in, by that I mean a lack of coordination between our eyes and the messages it interprets and the translating it to an activity.

Rather than getting heavily weighed down with the complicated science, the most important thing if you are concerned is to see you G.P. This is vital as several conditions mimic aspects of dementia but are treatable. For example a waterworks infection, a chest infection, dehydration or a poorly functioning thyroid gland can all to the untrained eye look like a dementia. When you talk to the doctor he will want to hear from you and the person affected what has been noticed and how it disrupts you on a day to day basis. They will want to take a blood sample to eliminate any of the conditions mentioned above. There would also be a physical examination of the person. The blood pressure would be checked and a urine sample may be asked for. Your doctor depending on the results may then recommend that the person is seen at Memory Clinic to try to establish further the probable cause of a dementia. Alzheimer's disease cannot be diagnosed, the consultant reaches the conclusion following the results of several tests, (which may include not only the history, blood tests, but also X-ray of the chest, CT scan and questionnaires) that the most probable cause for the memory problem is Alzheimer's'

The **early stages** of a dementia are defined by the person having a marked degree of memory difficulty and some loss of ability in coping with daily living activity due to impairment in one or more areas from the list above. This can vary hugely from person to person.

Alzheimer's is the most common condition which is a dementia. It is a progressive degenerative condition generally believed to belong to old age, this is a popular misconception. As stated above dementia is not a forgone conclusion of old age. There are several types of Alzheimer's some of which can affect people as young as 30 or 40 years of age. This is referred to as **Early Onset Dementia** and due to the young age of the person (under 65 yrs) brings a whole separate set of issues relating to where they are in life. For example their children may be at university or still at home. The mortgage is not yet paid and employment can be near impossible. It is not uncommon at the very early point of concern for people to go to their G.P presenting with features of depression. In time it becomes more evident that the cause for concern is due to **Early Onset Dementia.** Once again not all people who present with depressive type symptoms have a dementia, there can be many reasons. Only specific testing will determine the true nature of the complaint.

Alzheimer's is caused by the build up of tangles and plaques which leads to the destruction of the brain cells. All the elements from the list above may apply in varying degrees initially. Over a period of time all will apply.

Vascular Dementia is a common dementia which is not a normal part of aging. Whilst it is more common in older people it can happen at any age. For the brain to function it requires a good blood supply. The brain has a complex system of large and small blood routes. If there is a blockage or disruption to the blood supply being able to freely flow as it should, then death to the localised area of cells takes place. Whatever those cells are responsible for then becomes a function or thought failure. If we consider our washing machine as the body with numerous programmes controlled by a brain; and the pump as our heart, with the build up of limescale, we will in time experience a malfunction of the machine. The washing machine may still be able to operate some but not all programmes. The same is true of the brain.

So if the heart or blood vessels are faulty, or the blood is too thick for the heart to pump around the body, death of some brain cells, takes place. You may well hear the term "a stair case progression" used to describe the course of vascular dementia. This is because every time there is a disruption (mini bleed, T.I.A trans ischemic attack) to the blood flow then something the person could do before the incident they can no longer do after the incident. This may be recognising faces, tell the time on a digital watch or being able to comprehend alphabetical lists such as in a telephone book.

It is possible to have **Alzheimer's** and **Vascular Dementia.**

Lewy Body Dementia shares common features of both Alzheimer's disease and Parkinson's disease. It is more common in the over 65's but not unheard of in people who are younger. Lewy Bodies are very small spherical shaped protein deposits found in nerve cells. These deposits disrupt the normal functioning of the brain. It is a progressive condition comparable to Alzheimer's disease lasting several years (as long as no other medical condition interferes with the person's health.) The most common features of **Lewy Body Dementia** are that the ability to maintain attention and alertness is affected. Typically the memory is not affected to the same degree as in Alzheimer's. They will probably have difficulty in planning ahead and organising their thoughts. Physically there may be muscle stiffness and a tremor making skilled movements like eating and drinking without spillages a challenge. The loss of facial expression is also a feature making it seem as if the person is wearing a mask. This can be off putting for those around as they loose the clues of non verbal communication. It is quite usual for the person's abilities to vary during the course of the day, sometimes even from hour to hour. Visual hallucinations are a belief that you can see someone or something that is not actually there. It is not uncommon for people with **Lewy Bodies** to experience hallucinations especially of people or animals. Generally offering reassurance and distracting the person is more productive than entering into a heated discussion about whether or not what is being seen and experienced is real or not. I have known a gentleman with this condition who sees creepy crawlies coming out of his skin. It upsets his wife more than him as he seems to have a surreal detachment to the experience. Other features include having "funny turns"; they fall asleep easily and do not sleep well at night. They may also have falls for no apparent reason.

Frontal Temporal Lobe Dementia is any dementia causing damage to this area of the brain. It includes **Pick's Disease.** This is a progressive condition which occurs equally in men and women between the age of 40 -65 years. The difference between **Pick's Disease** and **Alzheimer's** is that in Pick's the frontal areas of the brain are affected in the early stages and in Alzheimer's it is the parietal lobe and temporal lobe. **Frontal Temporal Lobe Dementias** are progressive in nature. They are characterised by changes in the personality and changes in their social behaviour. Social etiquette goes out of the window as the person may start swearing in public and not see it as unacceptable. Possibly there will be impairment to the language used. Life for the carer and person affected may become chaotic as their judgement is damaged, they might go on spending sprees as they no longer comprehend the value of money and the process of paying for goods. It has been known for the police to be called as the shopkeeper believes the person to be a shop lifter. They are not doing it on purpose it is that they no longer have the ability to understand social laws. The rules do not apply to them. Along side this they lose the ability to rationalise the consequence of their actions and indeed may lose awareness to their personal safety, inviting strangers into the home. It can be exhausting for the carer and heart breakingly distressing as the person before the condition would never behave in such an erratic manner. It is possible to have the other side of the coin and the person becomes apathetic and depressed without expressing feelings of being sad. Their care in their personal appearance may becoming lacking causing upset to the carer, often with a sense of shame or embarrassment over their loved one's appearance. Obsessive actions which are not relevant to the situation may happen. One lady I met wanted to put face cream on but no longer recognised what was in any given container and took to repeatedly rubbing an abrasive bathroom cleaner on her face, (until the family realised what was going on and removed it.)

There are other conditions in which a dementia may become evident. If someone has had a significant **Head Injury** or a **Brain Tumour** they may experience symptoms of dementia. A sign is something that someone else can see, either visually, audibly, or by test results and a symptom is any indication of the condition perceived by the patient that the person tells you about. So pain is a symptom.

Parkinson's Disease.Multiple Sclerosis, Down's Syndrome and Huntingdon's Disease are all conditions whereby the patient could develop a dementia. As is **Korsakoff's syndrome** which is a chronic condition caused by sustained alcoholism, or may be metabolic or toxic in cause, including a deficiency in Vitamin B12 (thiamine). This is a difficult condition for the carer as the person has little if any insight into the cause of the condition. Life can be chaotic when they decide to have Christmas in the middle of august. If this group of people need to be admitted to hospital they are often nursed on a psycho-geriatric ward despite being in their 40's or 50's.

Memory loss in particular for recent events is apparent and the person is disorientated in their understanding of time and where they are.

It is not my intention to go into the medical aspects in depth, as each person while they will have a lot in common with others, they will also have differences. Your G.P or staff at the Memory Clinic/Community Mental Health Team/Older People's Mental Health Team (the titles vary around the country) will be better able to answer specific questions you have in light of the detailed knowledge they have of that person, and the medical investigations that have taken place in relation to the person's condition, both now and in the past.

All conditions have a wealth of available information about them, either in fact sheets, at local branches of relevant organisations or on the internet or at your local library. Your local Yellow Pages should have details of local branches of organisations.

Please look at the end of the book for useful contacts.

DAMAGE LIMITATION

All of us are wary of the unknown. Information gives us greater control. Planning for the unknowns the future may present is challenging. Often if we face the demons we can gain perspective. There are things we can do in time rather than finding it is too late. Arranging LASTING POWER OF ATTORNEY is one such thing. By taking legal advice now it can prevent distress in the future. It can bring peace of mind at an emotional time. You may strongly feel that this is a mile stone you are not yet ready to face. Let me ask you when is the right time?

By both of you taking legal advice now you can ensure that you and your loved ones know what your wishes are should it become necessary for them to have some control of your circumstances.

Arranging Lasting Power of Attorney on not just the person with a memory problem, but yourself too, allows their wishes, and yours to be explored and taken into account, whilst they have the capacity to do so. You ideally need people to have Lasting Power of Attorney on you as no one knows what the future health wise holds for any of us. It may seem to only be a good idea if you can see a condition which may affect decision making. This would stand true if your crystal ball guarantees that the unforeseen will not happen to you. Unfortunately as you already know life does not come with such guarantees. By doing this you are acknowledging with those around you a Plan B, in the event that it is needed.

Don't delay until tomorrow what can be done today. Age Concern has some useful fact sheets. Look in your Yellow Pages for a local firm of solicitors and make an appointment to discuss your personal requirements. Lasting Power of Attorney lasts until death at which point the Will takes over. It is not possible to go into any more detail here as everybody's financial and medical circumstances are different.

If you require a comprehensive booklet, below are details of how to access it;

Office of Public Guardian
Archway Tower
2 Junction Road
London N19 5SZ

Phone Number 0845 330 2900

Fax Number 020 7664 7705

E-mail customerservices@publicguardian.gsi.gov.uk

Website www.publicguardian.gov.uk

PREVENTION IS BETTER THAN THE CURE

It would be a positive step forward if you take time to consider the areas suggested below. By managing them now, you could prevent headaches it the future. All four areas could cause troublesome hurdles (if left to their own devices) somewhere later down the line.

Poor **Dental Hygiene** can become the cause of not wanting to eat if the dentures are ill fitting and not cleaned daily. It is painful to have a tomato pip stuck under a denture. Try to ensure regular check up's. The same goes for rotten or wobbly teeth; this can cause reluctance to eat. We all know how pointless and miserable toothache is.

Eye Care is another area to consider. Are the person's glasses clean? Are they fitting comfortable? Or do the rub behind the ears or on the bridge of the nose? Is the prescription still the right one? If the person has cataracts would surgery improve the quality of life? Regular check ups are again advisable.

If the person has a **hearing** difficulty this can lead to a lot of frustration all-round. Something else to be checked on a regular basis; It may be that they are prone to having wax accumulate. The nurse at your local doctors will be able to check for you and arrange for syringing if required.

Care of your life weary **feet** is the fourth area to keep a watchful eye on. If the socks are shrinking in the wash alongside the feet becoming swollen by the end of the day, it can restrict the circulation, which is not good. It is generally agreed that if you have diabetes that your toe nails should be seen to by a **chiropodist.** To prevent tripping up it is wise to ensure slippers have not become too loose. Many people notice a change in their shoe size, varying between mornings and later in the day. You should take this into account especially if you are purchasing footwear via a catalogue. Consider when the footwear is being worn and order the size accordingly. If the person is prone to their ankles becoming enlarged at the end of the day, they should sit with their feet up at various points through the day. They could also be encouraged to walk on a regular daily basis to aid the circulation. One golden rule is to not cross your legs when sitting!!!!

All of the above, by being taken charge of today we can Pave the Way towards reducing some unnecessary headaches tomorrow.

FINAL WORD

....

So dear carer we have reached the end of this first in a series of Carer Companion books. There is much for you to mull over. You now need time to take on board a whole array of new and possibly daunting concepts and practical tasks that need tending to. You need to allow yourself and the person you care for to come to terms, each of you at yours own pace, and adjust to a new place in your lives. I wish you and yours well and look forward to our paths crossing again in the next book Grasping The Nettle, where we will consider ways in coping with arising obstacles as well as a bit more about the workings of the brain. Take care of yourself.

Davina

USEFUL CONTACTS TO CONSIDER

ALZHEIMER'S SOCIETY
Devon House
58 St Katherine Way
London E1W 1JX

Helpline   0845 300 0336

Website   www.alzheimers.org.uk

AGE CONCERN ENGLAND
Age Concern Information Line
Linhay House
Ashburton
Devon TQ14 7UP

Information Line 0800 00 99 66
www.ageconcern.org.uk

CARERS UK
20 Great Dover Street
London SE1 4LX

Tel Number 020 7566 7637

Website www.carersuk.org

ATTENDANCE ALLOWANCE (if the person is over 65yrs) **/DISABILITY LIVING** (if the person is under 65 yrs) **ALLOWANCE CLAIM LINE**
Tel Number 08457 123456

BLUE BADGE SCHEME ring your local council (if you struggle with walking for any reason)

Ring your local council for a reduction in your council tax if you are in receipt of attendance allowance. If both husband and wife have physical disabilities and/or a memory problem then both are entitled to Attendance Allowance to meet their individual needs.

Headway
7 King Edward Court
King Edward Street
Nottingham NG1 1EW

Tel Number 115 9240800
Helpline 0808 800 2244
www.headway.org.uk

Parkinson's disease Society
National Office
215 Vauxhall Bridge Road
London SW1V 1EJ

Helpline 0808 800 0303
www.parkinsons.org.uk

Down's syndrome Association
Langdon Down Centre
2a Langdon Park
Teddington.   TW11 9PS

Helpline 0845 230 0372
www.downs-syndrome.org.uk

Huntingdon's Disease Association
Neurosupport Centre
Liverpool L3 8LR

Tel Number 0151 298 3298
www.hda.org.uk

All information correct at time of publishing.

Notes For Me

Notes For Me

Notes For Me

Notes For Me

Notes For Me

About the Author

Davina lives and works in Cambridgeshire. She is a qualified psychiatric nurse with a wealth of diverse experience. She has three sons, at one time the youngest pub landlady in Carmarthenshire. Spent 9 yrs working for Mencap in Wales. She has worked not only in the hospital setting but also in a care home. It is this wide range of work life and many of the carers she currently supports that has lead to this series being developed. Her philosophy lies in the belief of easy to understand bite sized and timely information being accessible to anyone with an interest, regardless of culture, age or lifestyle.

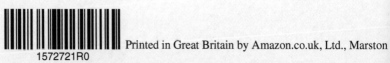
Printed in Great Britain by Amazon.co.uk, Ltd., Marston

1572721R0